Brain Foods

Eat your way to a better brain and live the
life you and your brain deserve

By: Dr. Chirag R. Patel
Board Certified Family Physician

Your Natural Youth

1202 N 75th Street, Suite 104
Downers Grove, IL 60516
www.YourNaturalYouth.com

DISCLAIMER

This book is not intended as medical advice. It is also not intended to prevent, diagnose, treat or cure disease. Instead the book is intended only to share the unofficial research and opinion of the author. The information is provided for educational purposes only, not as treatment instructions for any disease or ailment. Much of the book is a statement of opinion in areas where the facts are controversial or do not exist. The information in this book should not be considered any more valid than any other type of informal opinion.

The information was not written to replace the advice or care of a qualified health care professional. Be sure to check with your own qualified health care provider before beginning any protocols or procedures discussed in this book, or before stopping or altering any diet, lifestyle, or other therapies previously recommended to you by your health care provider.

The treatments described in this book may have side effects and carry other known and unknown risks and health hazards. The statements in this book have not been evaluated by the United States FDA. Use of the information in this book is at your own risk.

I dedicate this book to all my patients, their families, and all my family & friends for making me the physician, and person, I have become.

A Message For People Dedicated To Living Well and Living Long

Longevity. Who in their right minds wouldn't want to live a long, happy and fulfilling life? *To be able to help patients live well, caring for them and allowing them to enjoy life to its fullest and everything else it has to offer.* That is the unspoken mantra of every health care practitioner —or should be. Having been a physician for more than 10 years now, I know full well it has been mine. My name is Dr. Chirag R. Patel and I would love to provide you what my years of medicinal practice have taught me on living well and living long.

It has been my practice's goal (as well as my life's) to be able to provide my patients with the utmost service possible when it comes to caring for their health and well being. As a physician, I have always strived hard to turn this goal into "reality" at every given opportunity. I believe that reaching out, educating patients and empowering them to be responsibly active in caring for their health is part of a medical professional's duties. It is for this reason that I'm writing this book —allowing me to break the barriers of communication and be able to convey my message that living a long, happy and fulfilling life is all within your reach.

It is my deepest wish to be able to impart my knowledge on proper and responsible health care and its impact on how meaningful life can be. Let me guide you through the obstacles of aging with all the knowledge and resources that I have been able to gain over the years. There are so many easy things you can be doing today to start looking and feeling young. For the latest breaking news in longevity, visit me at www.YourNaturalYouth.com/sign-up and send me an email.

All the best,
Dr. Chirag R. Patel
drchiragpatel@yournaturalyouth.com

TABLE OF CONTENTS

Introduction.. 7

Chapter 1- The Foods Damaging Our Health 9

    High Fructose Corn Syrup 10

    Sodium... 13

    Artificial Sweeteners 17

    Energy Drinks 21

    Fast Food 26

    White Food.. 32

Chapter 2 -The Glycemic Index and Your Diet 37

    Utilizing the GI Ratings System in Your Diet....................... 38

    Is a Low GI Diet a Low-Carb Diet?...................................... 39

Chapter 3 - What to Include in Your New Diet 43

    Healthy Drinks.. 44

    Leafy Greens 48

    Fruit 52

    Spices 54

Recommended Reading 57

About the Author 61

INTRODUCTION

Navigating the murky waters of healthy eating and building the perfect diet is one of life's biggest challenges. Every day people eat foods that at first glance seem perfectly healthy. They buy food based on price or convenience, or in some cases food addictions, and very little thought is given to the way these foods affect our bodies. Foods have the power to heal and to harm, and yet we eat without a second thought.

For centuries medical professionals have understood the connection between nutrition and health. As Hippocrates said, "Let food be thy medicine." Even then food was seen as something that intended to provide more than just satisfaction from hunger. Over time we lost sight of this approach and learned to eat for reasons other than supplying our body with nutrition. This led to poor health, increased obesity rates, disease epidemics, and a society that is self-medicating with food. For many, food is a crutch, a comfort, and a social tool, but rarely these days is it viewed as a means of truly feeding the body what it needs to survive. In order for us to get healthy, we must once again learn to eat.

This might seem like the simplest thing in the world and yet, here we are, struggling every day to make the right food choices. Marketing and mistruths have muddled the meaning of what it means to make healthy food choices. Too much focus is placed on dieting and looking a certain way, and not enough emphasis is placed on caring for one's health. Food can heal, but you must first end the damage your current diet is causing.

Everyone has easy access to some of the unhealthiest foods in existence. These foods are cheap and plentiful. In some cases they are barely even foods. We are putting chemicals into our bodies that fill us up, but we are not getting the nourishment we need. We are poisoning our bodies with foods that might look and taste perfectly fine, but we do not realize the damage they are causing until it is too late.

We have access to tools and information that can help us make healthy changes in our diets, but we often resist the changes. Dietary changes require more than just a difference in our menus; they require a difference in our attitudes toward food, health, healing, and nourishment. We must alter our approach to eating, as well as the specific things we put into our mouths.

Once we have eliminated the dangers from our diets and opened our minds to a new approach to food, there are limitless options from which to choose. Filling our plates with delicious, natural, nutritious foods is one of the easiest things in the world to do once we are educated. Food can heal us from the inside out and help us lead better lives. It all starts with knowledge and a willingness to improve.

CHAPTER 1- THE FOODS DAMAGING OUR HEALTH

Everyone knows there are healthy foods and junk foods, but not as many people realize the effects these bad foods are actually having on our health. Making matters worse, there are a lot more junk foods out there than most people know. Foods mistakenly viewed as wholesome or appropriate to eat on a regular basis actually contain ingredients that are destroying our health.

To change your eating habits and improve your health with food, you must first understand what is causing you damage. Obviously, candy and cookies and chips are high on the list. These are commonly accepted as junk food and provide your body no nourishment. Not only are they junk food, they are filled with chemicals and preservatives that damage the body's cells. The junk foods we knew were harming us are causing even more damage than we realized.

In addition to known junk foods, many of the foods we consider healthy and wholesome contain these same chemicals and preservatives. Nobody thinks of bread, ketchup, peanut butter, juice, milk, cereal, or meat as junk food, but in many cases that is exactly what it is. Some foods start out harmless, but the manufacturers' effort to lengthen its shelf life or lower its cost damages the product. Other foods are actually not foods at all. They are developed in a lab, made to look, taste, and feel like familiar foods, and packaged and marketed to the public as perfectly safe. People serve these foods to their family everyday assuming they are nutritious and wholesome food options, but nothing could be further from the truth.

If you are ready to make changes in your diet and embark on a new, healthier lifestyle, your journey must first begin by learning about ingredients. To create a diet that will aid your body in growing stronger and healthier, you must read food labels and understand what foods promote health and what foods tear apart your body. Once you understand the ingredients that are damaging your body the most, you can begin to make changes and eliminate these dangerous foods.

HIGH FRUCTOSE CORN SYRUP

High fructose corn syrup or (HFCS) is a sweetening ingredient utilized for a variety of commercial foods, including soft drinks, juices, packaged bakery goods, cereal, breads, and snack foods. It is estimated that the average American consumes approximately 60 pounds of HFCS per year. It was introduced to the American food market in the mid-1970s and its use increased dramatically in the decade that followed. Many people draw a parallel between the introduction of HFCS and the skyrocketing rates of obesity that have occurred within the same time frame. Prior to the introduction of HFCS in 1970, obesity rates in the United States hovered around 15%. Today those rates are around 35% and expected to rise.

The dangers of high fructose corn syrup are controversial, but as more research is conducted people are beginning to accept there are risks associated with consuming this sweetener. Originally, high fructose corn syrup was billed as a natural, affordable alternative to table sugar and other sweeteners. The calorie content is approximately the same as table sugar and it is a convenient method for sweetening drinks and foods. Unfortunately, the convenience and cost savings is not worth the risk.

Although having similar chemical properties to table sugar, many believe that High fructose corn syrup is processed differently by the body compared to that of common sugar. Even those who believe HFCS is relatively safe acknowledge there is a problem with the amount of sugar in our diets. This is where HFCS becomes a problem across the board: it is hidden in many unexpected places, so even if it is safe in and of itself, massive consumption is not safe. If HFCS did not exist, it would be impossible to squeeze as much sugar as we do into our diets. In one way or another, HFCS absolutely plays a role in the incidences of obesity, diabetes, high triglycerides, and metabolic syndrome we see in modern society.

Studies Show HFCS Causes Weight Gain

Those who do not accept the safety of even limited amounts of HFCS cite studies showing the effects the product has on the brain. A Princeton study showed rats react differently to HFCS than they do to other sweeteners. When the rats were given HFCS they gained significantly more weight than when they were fed sugar, even if their total caloric intake remained the same.

The study also showed the rats gained greater amounts of body fat. The weight they gained from eating HFCS was pure fat, centered primarily in the middle, and led to an increase in triglycerides.

Naysayers of the study cite the delivery of the HFCS. A test conducted used rats that were given pure syrup, while human test subjects consumed food products with HFCS content. Unfortunately, this test study does little to prove that HFCS is safe and actually highlights the potential dangers. The rats ate far less HFCS than the average person consumes on a regular basis.

Similar outcomes occurred in studies involving HFCS. The first compared male rats that were given water mixed with HFCS and a standard diet of rat chow to rats given the same amount of food, but with water administered with table sugar. The first group of rats accumulated more weight compared to those that were given with table sugar in their water. The water solution contained half the concentration of HFCS than found in most soft drinks.

The second study took a long-term look at the effects of HFCS and obesity. The weight, body fat, and triglyceride levels of the study animals were followed and compared to a test group of rats fed only rat chow. The rats consuming HFCS experienced abnormal weight gain, an increase in triglycerides, and an increase in visceral fat in the belly. Both male and female rats were used in the study and the male rats showed a higher gain in size than females. Researchers noted the rats were not just gaining weight or getting fat, they were actually experiencing detrimental changes in their health related to obesity.

Chemical Structure and Manufacturing of HFCS

Researchers also believe they understand the reason for the rat's reactions in the studies. Both table sugar and HFCS contain fructose and glucose. However, table sugar is made up of equal amounts (50% and 50%) of both sugars, while HFCS contains 55% fructose and 42% glucose. The remaining 3% is saccharides, which are larger sugar molecules than glucose or fructose.

The manufacturing process for HFCS is also different than that of table sugar. HFCS contains free and unbound fructose molecules that are more easily absorbed in the body. These molecules do not have to go through the extra metabolic step like other sugars. In addition to its effect on metabolism and obesity, many medical experts believe HFCS is an addictive substance. Conspiracy theorists believe this was intentional, but even if it was not, it still makes a powerful statement about the control people relinquish to the food industry. The fructose in HFCS has a direct effect on the central nervous system. It is believed to cause a sensation of pleasure and trigger a craving for more HFCS. Some have compared it to alcohol, but without the depressive effects. HFCS gives you the pleasurable boost without the downside, essentially creating a substance more dangerous to our health than alcohol.

Should you eliminate HFCS from your diet? If you are concerned about your weight or your health, yes. Even if the current studies are disproven or further studies show the effects of HFCS are not as bad as originally thought, it is not worth the risk. The foods featuring HFCS are junk and there are much healthier options that taste just as great, if not better.

Many people find that by eliminating HFCS from their diet, their tolerance for sweet tastes decreases and they no longer enjoy the packaged, unhealthy products containing the sweetener. Some people even report improvements in general health, such as a reduction in headaches, stomach aches, and fatigue, though these are only anecdotal occurrences.

The bottom line is HFCS is not worth the risk and it should be one of the first things eliminated from your diet as you make health improvements. There is no reason why people need to consume the amount of sugar they have grown accustomed to eating, regardless of how it is delivered. By eliminating HFCS, you are cutting back on your overall sugar intake, creating space for healthier, more nutritious options.

SODIUM

Excess sodium is another problem in the standard American diet and the diets of those around the world accepting a Western style of eating. In addition to cooking with salt or using it as a condiment, salt is also hidden in a variety of unexpected places. Many people are not aware they are exceeding their daily sodium requirements. They Mayo Clinic estimates the average adult consumes at least twice as much sodium as she needs each day. Yes, people do need to consume a certain amount of sodium, but overdoing it can be very dangerous. Unfortunately, far too many people are exceeding their minimum and then some. They are headed down a dangerous road of poor health, compounded by the fact that high sodium levels are usually not the only problem for people with poor diets.

What is Considered Healthy Sodium Intake?

Sodium, much like sugar, occurs naturally in many different foods. If you are eating dairy, certain vegetables, and drinking water, you are likely meeting your minimum sodium requirements. For men and women between ages 10 and 50, the daily requirement is between 1500 and 2300 mg. After age 50 sodium limits should be reduced to 1300 mg and then to 1200 after age 70. Pre-adolescent children should limit their sodium intake to no more than 2200 mg.

Sodium requirements and limits are very specific for children. Children age birth to six months should consume approximately 120 mg of sodium per day. From seven months to one year 370 mg is appropriate. From one to three years old children should consume approximately 1000 mg per day and from age four to eight, the appropriate amount is 1200 mg. For the most part, children over the age of one should be limited to no more than 1900 mg of sodium per day.

It can be confusing for some people to understand why something considered so unhealthy is actually a necessary part of a healthy diet. If something is unhealthy, it should be eliminated right? Not in this case. Sodium is necessary for good health and is responsible for the health of the heart, brain, bones, and muscles. Sodium also provides electrolytes, keeping cells balanced and protected. In moderation, sodium keeps the body functioning and healthy. The problem occurs when sodium is eaten in excess. Too much of a good thing is no longer a good thing.

The best way to maintain healthy sodium levels without overdoing it is to consume your daily required sodium in natural foods. If you are adding table salt to your food or eating a lot of processed, preserved, or so-called convenience foods, you are likely eating too much sodium. Foods considered the biggest sodium bombs include lunch meat, bacon, and certain condiments. Believe it or not salt substitutes can also be dangerous, mainly because they force your kidneys to work harder than they should. If you have a sodium problem, begin by eliminating these items from your diet. Cut back to only the natural sources of sodium and build from there, if necessary. This adjustment can take time and you will need to research the sodium in natural foods, but revamping your diet and fixing an excess sodium problem can save your life.

Dangers of Sodium

Exceeding maximum sodium levels once in a while is not likely to cause a great deal of harm if you are healthy otherwise. Unfortunately, people are regularly exceeding these amounts, even when they believe their diets are fairly healthy. Over time, these mistakes can have devastating results.

Too much sodium leads to fluid buildup which causes numerous problems. On the mild side, fluid retention causes you to look bloated and overweight, even if you are within a healthy weight range. On the other end of the spectrum, fluid retention can be a serious problem for people with congestive heart failure, or problems with their kidneys or liver.

Blood pressure is another major concern for those consuming too much sodium. If you are prone to high blood pressure, sodium will cause it to spike. If you currently have healthy blood pressure, long-term excessive consumption of sodium can cause high blood pressure. Excessive sodium can also have a negative effect on asthma, stomach cancer, kidney stones, and Alzheimer's disease. Some health experts even believe too much sodium can affect intelligence and long- and short-term memory.

Chronically exceeding maximum sodium recommendations can also lead to an imbalance between sodium and potassium in the body's cells. When this occurs, cell health is damaged, weakening overall health and possibly triggering the development of specific diseases.

Remember, your body is comprised of cells. When these cells are damaged and unhealthy, you are damaged and unhealthy. Keeping your cells healthy is an important part of reducing your risk for disease and feeling your best in the here and now.

The Sodium Problem We All Face

Despite the knowledge that is out there concerning the dangers of high sodium levels, people still exceed their recommended daily allowance every day. As a matter of fact, the connection between too much salt, high blood pressure, and poor heart health is one of the most well-known of all the food related health concerns. Even people who understand very little about how their diet affects their health know too much salt is bad for them. Yet very little changes and as a society, we continue to consume too much salt.

Why is this? The problem likely has several components. For starters, salt is hidden in a variety of foods. Most people assume gooey sweets are unhealthy because of their sugar content, but few guess these treats are loaded with salt. The same is true for things seemingly innocent, such as loaves of bread, bottles of ketchup, or a simple ham sandwich. In order to keep sodium levels in a healthy range, people must be diligent about reading labels and educating themselves.

Another part of the problem is habit. Though salt is not considered as addictive as sugar, it is a popular craving. Ask anyone what their most common cravings are and they will likely answer either sugary or salty treats. There is something appealing about munching on salty snacks, even if we know they are unhealthy.

Finally, our lack of time is a problem. People are busier than ever with tasks that do not revolve around nutrition and preparing healthy meals. When pressed for time, it is easier to grab prepared foods. Some of these are fast food options that can be eaten on the go, but sit-down meals in restaurants can also be a problem. Do not assume that because you are dining in at a restaurant you are being served a healthy meal that is low in sodium. As a matter of fact, these meals are some of the worst culprits when it comes to salt. This is partly because serving sizes are huge, partly because the food must be preserved for long periods of time, and partly because we have developed a taste for high salt foods. Most people notice within just a few days of cutting back on sodium, their tolerance for salty foods decreases.

If diet improvements are a goal, sodium is a great place to start. Even if you are not suffering from high blood pressure or any other health afflictions related to salt, it is a good idea to reduce your sodium intake. In doing so, you will likely make secondary improvements in your diet, too.

ARTIFICIAL SWEETENERS

A common mistake those who are new to dieting and healthy eating make is to assume that since sugar is bad, artificial sugar must be fine. It is free of calories and is billed as "safe" by the FDA. Most people reason that if it is so readily available, it will not cause harm. Unfortunately, nothing is further from the truth. Not only are artificial sweeteners dangerous, they just do not work. Some believe they actually have the exact opposite effect users want: they lead to weight gain.

So how can something dangerous and ineffective make it into our food when government regulations claim to control these things? In the case of artificial sweeteners, they use semantic loopholes. Artificial sweeteners fall into the category of foods that are "Generally Recognized as Safe" (GRAS). The general safety is determined by scientists employed by the government. (As a side note, some believe there are conflicts of interest when it comes to getting foods and medications approved as safe. The details are too

17

lengthy to go into here, but it is worth looking into if you are concerned about food and drug safety.)

Artificial sweeteners fall into a category known as non-nutritive sweeteners. They were invented in the 1950s, but it was actually by accident that researchers realized the chemicals created could be used to sweeten foods. Since then, they have been used as a way to reduce both the calories in and the cost of making certain foods. The artificial sweetener market gradually increased until it reached its boom around the turn of the Twenty-first century. More than 6,000 new products were introduced to the market featuring artificial sweeteners between 1996 and 2006.

There are multiple approved artificial sweeteners. Safety guidelines include an acceptable daily intake before health risks become a problem. So right out of the gate, the FDA is admitting it is possible for these substances to be dangerous. Granted, everything can be dangerous if consumed to excess. However, aside from eliminating calories, artificial sweeteners provide no nutritive benefits. Basically, nature never intended humans to eat something like this and each of the artificial sweeteners comes with its own unique blend of dangers.

Saccharin

Saccharin was removed from the official list of potential carcinogens in 1997. However, doubts still remain about saccharin and many health experts believed removing it from the list gave the public a false sense of security. In addition to concerns about saccharin being a carcinogen, there are also concerns about allergies. People unable to tolerate sulfa drugs can react badly to saccharin and experience headaches, skin irritations, diarrhea, and difficulty breathing. Most astonishing is saccharin's use in some baby formulas. It is known to cause muscle dysfunction and irritability in infants, but the FDA does not believe there is sufficient evidence to issue an official warning.

Aspartame

Aspartame is one of the better known controversial ingredients. Even people who spend relatively little time educating themselves about food safety and health likely know there are concerns about aspartame. Though some concerns about the artificial sweetener might be hyperbole, there are certain facts about aspartame that are agreed upon by most medical professionals. The way in which aspartame is digested in one concern. Some artificial sweeteners enter and exit the body in the same form. Aspartame, on the other hand, is metabolized by the body, which essentially means it can do more damage.

There is such a thing as "aspartame disease". The description was coined by author H.J. Roberts, MD and refers to the negative reactions people have when they ingest aspartame. Dr. Roberts lists symptoms such as headaches, vomiting, nausea, mood changes, dizziness, abdominal pain and cramping, diarrhea, memory loss, fatigue, and seizures. Some also believe that aspartame consumption is associated with fibromyalgia, joint pain, depression, anxiety, multiple sclerosis, lupus, and cancer. Cancer, headaches, and depression all have at least one study backing up their connection. The first study that linked brain tumors in rats with aspartame was later challenged by a French and Italian study disproving the link between cancers in humans and aspartame. Despite these latest findings, research continues to determine if there is a link.

One study that did prove a theory true was that of linking aspartame to increased hunger. Basically, substituting so-called sugar free foods to lose weight can basically lead to weight gain. The study followed 14 dieters who consumed diet soft drinks. The dieters drinking the diet drinks consumed just as many calories as they would have drinking regular soda and in some cases, they consumed even more calories than usual.

Sucralose

Sucralose is the sweetener that when listed on an ingredient list might appear to be regular sugar, but it is not. It is actually nothing like sugar and was discovered during an experiment to develop a new pesticide. Sucralose alters sugar by treating it with a myriad of noxious sounding chemicals. One of the products that utilize sucralose actually features a warning that states, "Although sucralose has a structure like sugar and a sugar-like taste, it is not natural." One of the ingredients used to treat sugar when making sucralose is chlorine. This is a proven carcinogen. It should also be noted that no long-term studies have been conducted on sucralose.

In addition to having a disturbing manufacturing process, sucralose is not even a calorie-free sweetener. A cup of the artificial sweetener containing sucralose has nearly 100 calories. It is 600 times sweeter than natural sugar, so only a small amount of it is needed to achieve the desired effect. When flavoring iced tea or coffee with sucralose, it is unlikely a large enough amount would be used to create a significant calorie intake. However, research has shown that some people consume up to a cup of sucralose per day when so-called diet foods are taken into account. Dieters might be consuming more than 100 unintended calories per day if they are eating foods sweetened with sucralose.

The problems do not end there. Studies have also shown that sucralose affects the absorption of medication in rats. The same studies have been performed on humans with varying results. Further studies are planned to determine the accuracy of previous findings, but in the meantime, people are consuming sucralose every day.

Neotame

Neotame is the least recognized of the artificial sweeteners. The manufacturers of neotame claim it is completely safe and point to multiple studies supporting their claims. Others believe, though, neotame could still pose long-term danger. The sweetener is similar to aspartame, so one can assume there are also similar risks.

The bottom line is nobody is absolutely sure artificial sweeteners are directly related to health problems. The trouble is they also are not sure if the sweeteners are safe. What this means is that people concerned about their health should err on the side of caution. Regarding artificial sweeteners this is an easy task. Replace artificial sweeteners with other options. This will include a bit of cutting back overall on certain foods, but you still have plenty of options. There are natural calorie-free sweeteners, such as stevia. You can also continue to eat regular sugar, but do so in moderation. Honey is another option, though it is not calorie free. There are few foods as easy to eliminate from your diet as artificial sweeteners, so it is a great place to start if you want to make health improvements and feed your brain and body what is really needs.

ENERGY DRINKS

Energy drinks continue to grow in popularity. These are not drinks intended for after workouts. Those are meant to rehydrate you and balance electrolytes, while energy drinks are intended to boost energy. Pre-workout drinks have a number of weaknesses, but they are not as dangerous as energy drinks. Energy drinks are intended to boost your energy for a few hours at a time. In the past, people would choose soda or coffee for this. Not healthy choices, but again, not as bad as energy drinks. If you are a frequent user of energy drinks or you have been tempted to grab one of these drinks on an afternoon that is just dragging by, there are several things you need to know.

Though they are perfectly legal and sold in most stores that sell drinks, snacks, and food, energy drinks are dangerous. Not only are they packed with ingredients that are harmful, they can actually trigger serious medical reactions, including heart attack and stroke. An Australian study showed that drinking energy drinks increases the risk of these cardiovascular issues. It is actually the energy companies that market their drinks as completely safe and labeling regulations that leave loopholes, making it possible for the companies to make bold claims about the health benefits of their drinks. Ask most medical professionals how they feel about energy drinks and they will say they are concerned and that the drinks should include clear labels about their risks. At the least, there should be further studies conducted on the drinks before they are deemed safe commercially.

The energy drink market is booming. The drinks are consumed by people in the morning to get revved up, before workouts, during late nights working or out on the town, and by kids wanting a boost throughout their school day. Some estimates place the earnings for energy drinks at more than $5 billion per year. For a small portion of the population, energy drinks are safe. They can be consumed without consequence, even though most of the commercially sold brands are not all that nutritious. Unfortunately, energy drinks have proven harmful to people suffering from specific conditions. Anyone with anxiety or any other nervous disorder can have a bad reaction to energy drinks. The drinks have even been known to trigger episodes for people with anxiety disorders.

It should come as no surprise that energy drinks are loaded with caffeine. Some feature no more than a few cups of coffee, but others are loaded with the stimulant. Energy drinks provide an even bigger boost than the other beverages because the caffeine is paired with vitamins and herbs. Sounds healthy? It is meant to, but these are herbs mixed together in ways that can be dangerous. Chances are your energy drink is coming from a can at the local supermarket or convenience store and not an experienced herbalist. To make matters even worse and really distinguish these drinks from other energy boosting solutions, these drinks are packed with sugar.

The sugar level in the drinks are so intense researchers have reported that a person's blood actually becomes sticky after drinking one of the most popular brands of these drinks. This is a warning sign of cardiovascular problems. As one of the leading killers of Americans, health researchers are very familiar with the signs and symptoms associated with heart attacks and strokes. Though many of the incidences are related to obesity and genetics, energy drinks increase the likelihood of a problem. If you are already at risk, you are increasing your chances of having a cardiovascular incident. If you have no risks, you are creating them by drinking energy drinks.

Caffeine

As mentioned earlier, the caffeine levels in energy drinks vary a great deal. Some are comparable to soda and coffee, while others have as much as 15 times the amount of caffeine found in popular sodas. Unfortunately, there are no warnings about these caffeine levels. Sodas label whether they are caffeinated and have actually turned their non-caffeinated products into powerful players in their product lines. Unfortunately, this is not the case for energy drinks. Some energy drinks contain up to 500 mg of caffeine, but have little warning about the content. In comparison, the average soda has about 35 mg and a cup of coffee has about 100 mg.

The other thing that troubles health professionals about energy drinks is that they are not marketed the same way as coffee and soda. Most people understand soda is junk food and coffee is an indulgence. There are a few health benefits to drinking some coffees, but you need to closely monitor your intake to limit the side effects. Energy drinks, on the other hand, are marketed as health or dietary supplements. This eliminates the need to follow FDA regulations regarding caffeine content. In soda, coffee, and a number of other beverages, the limit is 71 mg per 12 oz. Since energy drinks are supplements, the regulations do not apply. Even worse, the public is not educated. Someone might know the FDA has set a caffeine limit for beverages, but not realize that energy drinks do not fall under the same standards.

Other Side Effects

In addition to the problems related to caffeine levels in energy drinks, there are a number of other health risks associated with the beverages. Most dental health professionals agree that consuming energy drinks causes tooth decay. Obviously, this is related to the sugar content. A study published in General Dentistry, showed that energy drinks erode tooth enamel more than sodas and sports drinks.

Energy drinks can also cause heart palpitations and headaches. Anyone who has ever consumed too many cups of coffee knows what it feels like when too much caffeine is in the system. This usually takes three or four or more cups of coffee, but these same effects can occur with just one energy drink. One study showed that 22% of college aged adults drinking energy drinks experienced headaches and 19% experienced heart palpitations.

Energy drinks also seem to lower a person's inhibitions. Long-term studies have shown that people consuming more than six energy drinks per month are more likely to smoke cigarettes, engage in physical violence, and abuse prescription and illicit drugs. Some of the drinks even feature drug-related names. Adolescent and young adult drinkers, the target market for energy drinks, both report experiencing energy crashes throughout the week. Up to 29% of one study's participants stated they experienced jolts and crashes of energy, even when not directly related to consuming the drinks.

Mixing energy drinks with alcohol is a popular practice for young adult drinkers. They combine energy drinks with hard liquor, creating an up-all-night, hyperactive intoxicated state. Mixing energy drinks with alcohol impairs your perception more than alcohol alone. The energy boost can lead to a belief that you are less intoxicated than you are in reality, which leads to bad judgment and the reasoning that it is alright to continue drinking, even when you are long past the point of inebriation. A Wake Forest study even showed this risky combination of alcohol and energy drinks led to a higher risk of physical injury.

Energy Drink Consumption Leads to Death

Energy crashes and alcohol impairment might seem minor to some people, especially teens and young adults. Many reason the jolt is worth the crash, especially if a night of fun is on the agenda or an all-night cram session is needed. Furthermore, if drinkers choose not to mix the beverages with alcohol, they eliminate the risks associated with the combination. However, they are by no means in the clear when it comes to energy drink related risks.

Researchers point out that no long-term studies have been performed on energy drinks. It is believed these drinks affect brain function over the long haul, but it will take years to scientifically prove these theories. We are basically dealing with the first generation of energy drink consumers, so it could be a few decades before we see the long-term effects.

There have been four documented cases of caffeine-related deaths in conjunction with energy drink consumption. There have also been five cases of seizures. A young man in his late 20s experienced cardiac arrest after consuming an energy drink during a day of motocross. An 18 year old man died during a game of basketball after consuming two pre-game energy drinks. There have also been four diagnosed cases of mania in instances when those suffering from bipolar disorder drank an energy beverage. That is something else to keep in mind: if you are in perfect health, some of these risks might seem minor. However, if you suffer from even mild conditions, energy drinks can have a profound effect. And for some, fatal effects are possible.

Some researchers believe energy drinks also play a role in the development of insulin resistance and diabetes. With the high sugar content in the beverages, this is no surprise. No amount of enhanced athletic performance or metabolic increase is worth the risk of diabetes or heart disease. In reality, the proclamation of enhanced athletic performance is actually laughable. The drinks are filled with sugar and caffeine, both of which contribute to dehydration. Drinking an energy drink while working out is actually worse than drinking nothing at all during intense physical activity. Caffeine might improve muscle performance, but it is absolutely not worth the risk when delivered in such high quantities. Any benefit you might experience is far outweighed by the limitations and risks.

There are absolutely no health benefits to consuming energy drinks, no matter what the label might state. Even when these drinks are fortified with vitamins or energy-boosting herbs, the positive effects that would come from these items are canceled when taken in this form. You are better off drinking water and speaking with an experienced herbalist if you are interested in supplementing with herbs to boost your energy.

FAST FOOD

Entire books and movies are dedicated to the damage fast food has caused our country. Many health professionals believe it is the single biggest contributor to our current health crisis. What makes it even worse is that children are targeted in marketing plans and they eat fast food without a second thought. Childhood and adolescence is a time for risk taking and feeling invincible, but children do not even realize they are taking risks when eating fast food. In order for people to truly understand the risks associated with eating these cheap, convenient meals, they must understand all of the risks. The problem is much worse than just eating junk food or splurging on a quick treat from the drive-thru.

Fast Food has a High Fat Content

Just about anything you order from any fast food menu is going to be loaded with fat. Some restaurants have begun offering "healthier" choices, which is of course relative to the other garbage on the menu. For the most part, though, anything you order from a fast food establishment is filled with cholesterol.

The reason fast food is so high in cholesterol is because of the cooking oil used to prepare the foods. Fast food restaurants use the cheapest preparation option which is hydrogenated cooking oil. It has been scientifically altered to lengthen its shelf life, but these changes make it extremely dangerous. It is because of this oil the foods sold at these restaurants are loaded with trans fat. The body does not recognize trans fat as a food during digestion and stores it as fat cells, which lead to clogged arteries. You have probably heard about some restaurants banning trans fats, but be careful with these so-called health claims. A product does not need to be completely free of trans fats for it to be called trans fat free.

High Sugar Content

Fast food is often packed with sugar. Even if the individual food items you order are not sugary, they are typically packaged with a beverage. This means along with your unhealthy food you are getting a soda or novelty beverage containing HFCS or a diet beverage containing aspartame. No matter how you slice it, you are swallowing a whole lot of extra calories when grabbing a quick fast food meal. When you factor in the side orders, the bread, and the condiments, you increase the sugar and HFCS content even more.

This is problematic for two reasons. First, upping your sugar intake increases the calories you consume. In many cases people do not even realize how many more calories they are eating when dining on a fast food meal. For the amount of food you get and certainly the amount of nutrition, the calorie load is astronomical.

The other problem is the chemicals you are putting into your body. HFCS is not only high in calories, it is dangerous. And do not assume if you forego a beverage you are avoiding HFCS. It shows up in hamburger buns, condiments, and side dishes.

Lacking Nutritional Value

With all of the bad stuff fast food features, you would think there would be at least a few good things in it. It is jam-packed with everything that will kill you! Unfortunately, it is also lacking everything that offers any nutritional value. There is absolutely no health trade-off when you eat fast food. All you are doing is filling empty space, so you might not feel hungry for a few hours but your body is actually starving. When you consistently eat food lacking in nutrients, your hunger flares up faster than usual. The hungrier you are the more you will eat, which leads to overeating. As if one bad fast food meal was not enough, you are going to want two or three extra meals each day to make up for your nutrient deficiency.

There are also some who believe fast food is addictive. A study conducted at Princeton University showed that rats given fast food showed symptoms of addiction and withdraw. Scientists believe their brains experienced neuro-chemical changes that were similar to using narcotics. The changes were found in the dopamine and opiate receptors in the brain. Other studies have shown that eating fast food triggers pleasure centers in the brain, similar to what would occur if a person took heroin. The fast food industry continues to deny their food is addictive, but anecdotal proof shows otherwise. Do you know someone who indulges in fast food? Chances are it is not something they do only once or twice a year.

Low Quality Ingredients

One of the reasons fast food continues to be a successful industry is because the food is considered cheap. Now, when you sit down and plan a vegetarian meal with healthy foods, this is not always the case.

However, running through a drive-thru for a $6 fast food meal seems cheap at the time. This is especially true if you are used to buying large amounts of meat from the supermarket. The reason fast food restaurants are able to serve foods that should be expensive is because they use such low quality ingredients.

The fast food industry has drastically altered the slaughter and meat packing industry. In order to make a profit, they needed to find the cheapest way to get meat into people. The best way for them to cut costs is at the beginning of the process. This means the food that is served to you comes from abused animals living in poor conditions and slaughtered in an equally bad environment. The food you are eating when dining at a fast food restaurant is downright disgusting.

Unsafe Preparation

As if the food arriving at the restaurant were not bad enough, the process of preparing the food puts your health at even greater risk. Most fast food restaurants employ low-paid, relatively young employees. There are plenty of hard working people in the industry, but you also run a risk of having your food cooked by someone who is inexperienced with food safety or resentful of having to work in the industry. Too many times food slips through the cracks and makes it into your body, even though it is spoiled, undercooked, or riddled with disease.

The only way to avoid the dangers of fast food is to never eat it. Even an occasional fast food meal puts you at risk. There are far too many healthier, quick, and inexpensive options for dining to risk eating fast food. Instead of running through the drive-thru on the way home, stop at the supermarket or deli and grab a fruit salad and whole wheat crackers. A few containers of frozen or chopped veggies can be mixed with quinoa or brown rice for a stir fry. If you are going to splurge, try a take-out vegetarian option from your favorite restaurant. Vegetable based dishes are not as expensive as other options and ordering take-out saves on drinks and a tip.

If you are looking for an easy way to improve your diet, eliminate fast food. It is the easiest thing in the world you can do and it will make a tremendous difference in your health.

Fried Food

Many of the foods served at fast food restaurants are fried, but these establishments are not the only places you can get fried food. It is also important to realize that just because foods do not have that signature golden-brown batter covering them does not mean they are not fried during preparation. Frying food in oil creates a number of problems. Not only is it generally unhealthy because of the high fat content, it also changes the chemical structure of food. This means that frying normally healthy foods leaves you with an altered food that no longer has any nutritional value.

Trans Fat

The other problem with deep frying is that restaurant cooks and people frying at home typically use the oil several times. It heats and cools three or more times before it is deemed dirty enough to replace. The oil goes from a liquid to a solid and back again several times through partial hydrogenation. This makes the oil even more dangerous because it increases a compound in the oil called HNE. HNE is better known as trans fat. It occurs in high levels in polyunsaturated oils that contain linoleic acid. These are the most common oils used in fast food restaurants and include corn, canola, soybean, and sunflower. HNE only exists in plant oils, not in animal fat. Foods such as margarine, pies, some bread, chips, crackers, cookies, and doughnuts are the biggest culprits when it comes to trans fatty food.

Trans fats are being phased out in some places, but continue to be used frequently, especially in restaurants in certain parts of the country. There are alternatives, but they are more expensive, which is why restaurants opt for the cheaper trans fat option. Exposure to trans fat is linked to cardiovascular disease, Huntington's disease, stroke, Parkinson's, Alzheimer's disease, liver ailments, and cancer.

Even oils that are typically considered healthy, such as olive oil, might become dangerous when heated. All liquid oils undergo oxidative damage when heated, so do not assume that something cooked in healthy oil is safe. You are always better off consuming healthy oils cold.

There are a number of risks associated with eating fried foods and better understanding these risks discourages you from eating this way. When you know what you are doing to your body with unhealthy food you are more likely to opt for healthier alternatives. Avoiding restaurant food is one of the best ways you can prevent exposure to reheated plant oils. If you do dine out, ask about the oils used in preparation. Order sautéed foods if you must get foods cooked in oil and request that the chef sauté the food at no more than a moderate temperature.

Avoid packaged snacks and treats. Foods such as potato chips and snack cakes are prepared with trans fat oil. Shop for cold pressed oils when buying oil to use at home and do not heat these oils for cooking. Sprinkling raw and steamed vegetables with cold pressed oils is a healthy way to consume your needed fat, but cooking those oils negates the health benefits. If you must cook with oil at home, choose stable oils, such as coconut oil. It has a number of healthy benefits and does not change when heated at high temperatures. Ideally though, you want to avoid fried foods as much as possible.

The consumption of fried foods is quickly becoming one of the country's worst health risks. Experts believe that as many as 30,000 premature deaths each year are caused by a diet high in trans fat. Some believe that the elimination of margarine would be enough to cut back on more than 6,000 heart attacks each year. Though you have likely learned otherwise at some point, margarine is far worse than regular butter. There is also a financial impact to altering how we eat fat. The FDA estimates that finding a healthier way to make cookies and crackers would save nearly 60 billion dollars in health care costs over the next two decades. In addition to just making you fat, trans fat boost LDL cholesterol and insulin levels, and reduces HDL cholesterol.

Making Improvements

There are a few rules you can follow to make your decisions about oils and fats easier. Begin by eliminating the worst culprits. These are the foods you already know are unhealthy if you have begun making diet changes. The list includes margarine, baked goods unless you make them yourself, potato and corn chips, shortening, many salad dressings, and some breakfast cereals. Your goal is not necessarily to lower your overall fat intake, but to limit saturated fat and eliminate trans fat. Animal fats, such as meat and dairy, should only be a small portion of your diet, if any.

When consuming oil, remember the softer the better and liquid is best. Stick butters and margarines are worse than tub options, and bottled liquid oils are better than tubs. Chances are if you are concerned about your health enough to make changes and learn how to eat better, you are already to the point of consuming only healthy oils. However, you need to look for hidden dangers in many packaged and restaurant foods.

WHITE FOOD

Learning everything you need to know about healthy eating and protecting your body from dietary harm is challenging. It takes time and at times it feels overwhelming. This is why using a few healthy eating rules can help you make improvements quickly, as you learn all of the ins and outs of nutrition. One of the best rules to implement when you are new to healthy eating is the "no white food" rule. With only a few exceptions, such as white beans and cauliflower, eliminating white food from your diet can make a world of difference. This is because most white foods are made with white sugar and white flour. White flour is wheat that has been refined and bleached. It is void of nutritional value and actually contains chemicals that harm your health.

White flour uses only a portion of the whole grain of wheat. Grains of wheat, or wheat berries, have three layers. The bran layer is the hard outer shell where the fiber is contained. The endosperm is the largest part of the grain and is made up of mostly starch. The germ is the embryo of the grain, loaded with nutrients and capable of sprouting a new wheat plant. Only the endosperm is used in white flour. That's right: ONLY the worst part of the wheat grain is used for making white bread, so you are consuming bread void of all its nutritional value! True whole wheat flour contains all three parts of the grain and is always your better choice.

Some experts believe the process to create white flour essentially turns it into white sugar. The wheat grains are exposed to high-temperatures and high-speed rollers when ground and used for mass production. This eliminates nearly all of the vitamin E content, half the calcium and unsaturated fatty acids, 70% of the phosphorous, 80% of the iron, and 90% of the magnesium. At least half of the B vitamins are also eliminated.

Chemical Danger

Unfortunately, the problem is not only the way in which the wheat is processed. There are also problems with how the ingredients for bread are grown. According to many health experts, buying a loaf of white bread is like buying a loaf of dangerous pesticides. The bread is made from wheat seeds that have been treated with a fungicide chemical before they are even planted in the ground. Once the wheat begins to grow, the crops are sprayed with more pesticide and hormones. Once harvested, the wheat is stored in bins that have been sprayed to kill bugs. Finally, the wheat is given a final spray of pesticide to kill any super-strong pests that might have survived the previous treatments.

Guess what? All of these chemicals intended to kill life do not go away once the wheat is turned into bread. The only way you are guaranteed a healthy loaf of bread is to purchase organic products that provide information about the growing process of the ingredients or to bake your own bread using chemical-free, whole grain flour.

Worse, MORE chemicals are added during the manufacturing process! Flour should be aged before it is used in baking, but this is no longer an option in the commercial, mass-production industry. Instead, chlorine oxide is used to age, bleach, and oxidize the flour. Health experts believe the chlorine oxide interacts with the proteins in flour to produce alloxan. Alloxan has been used to create diabetes in lab animals in order to test diabetes treatments on the animals. Think about that for a moment: the exact compound used to trigger diabetes in an animal intentionally is fed to another animal (us!) in loaves of bread. Is this something you want to use to make a sandwich? In addition to the chlorine oxide, flour is also exposed to nitrogen oxide, benzoyl peroxide, and nitrosyl during the milling process.

How does your body react to these chemicals and the lack of nutrition in white four? First, it gains weight because you are feeding it empty calories. Like many "foods" void of nutrition, you are filling your stomach with stuff, but your body thinks it is starving. It shows this through hunger, so you continue to eat never satisfying your body's needs, but consuming more and more calories.

White flour has also been shown to raise cholesterol, interfere with the body's use of essential fatty acids, and upset insulin levels. The body breaks white flour down into sugar and is unable to tell the difference between eating a slice of white bread and eating several tablespoons of sugar. White flour has also been shown to cause constipation. This means all of the toxins you are eating stick around in your body much longer, causing even more damage.

What Can You Do?

Obviously, avoid white flour. Opt instead for whole grain products and read labels carefully. There are plenty of tricks used in the wheat industry to make you think white flour is OK. "Enriched white flour," "enriched wheat flour," and white bread claiming to be fortified with nutrients are all garbage. You need to choose bread that lists "whole grain flour" as its first ingredient. You can also swap out wheat flour with rye and oat flours, almond meal, brown rice flour, or millet flour. Spouted breads are a great option because you know they contain all of the nutrition originally found in the wheat berry.

Going wheat-free is also an option. For those with gluten sensitivities, wheat-free is the only option, but this is not a great idea for those without the sensitivity. You should not cut something nutritious out of your diet unless absolutely necessary. Like most diet improvements, begin making swaps when you shop for food. Read labels, look for the highest quality ingredients, and educate yourself about how products affect your health.

Chapter 2 - The Glycemic Index and Your Diet

One of the tools you can use to improve your diet is the glycemic index (GI). It is a method for ranking the carbohydrates in certain foods. Foods are ranked from 0 to 100 based on their effect on the body's blood sugar level. Foods that are considered high in glycemic index are digested quickly and create a fluctuation in blood sugar levels. Low GI foods digest slowly and gradually increase blood sugar levels. In general, low GI foods are better for you.

Some medical professionals recommend low GI diets to improve health, lose weight, or manage health conditions, such as diabetes. Low GI diets improve both glucose and lipid levels, which is helpful for both types 1 and 2 diabetes. In addition to controlling blood sugar, low GI diets also control hunger, which helps with weight loss.

There is a great deal of scientific evidence backing up the benefits of low GI diets. A study from the Harvard School of Public Health shows that low GI diets reduce the risks of diabetes and coronary heart disease. The World Health Organization has also recognized the benefits of low GI diets.

Determining a food's GI rating is complicated, so the average person uses the official ratings system. GI ratings were developed by feeding foods to subjects and testing their blood. Blood sugar levels are tested for a period of two hours following consumption of a specific food and a blood sugar curve of measurements is recorded. The GI is then calculated by multiplying the numbers associated with the curve by 100. Obviously, this is a very scientific process which is not necessary to repeat again and again. Once a food's GI rating is established, it remains the same regardless of the amount of food and who is consuming it.

GI rating is growing in popularity as a means of determining a food's nutritional value. Some countries, such as Australia, list a food's GI rating on its packaging. Some organizations prefer that foods feature carbohydrate content instead of GI value.

UTILIZING THE GI RATINGS SYSTEM IN YOUR DIET

If you are interested in using GI ratings as a guide for improving your diet, there are a few things you should understand. First, you do not need to eat only low GI foods to see results. The effects of low GI foods carry into future meals. This means that the glycemic impact of foods is affected by foods eaten hours earlier. Guidelines encourage eating one low GI meal per day to keep blood sugar levels stable. It will not harm you to focus on eating low GI foods, but you do not have to limit your diet that drastically. You can even combine high and low GI foods to achieve a medium GI rating.

One of the things about GI rating that might be hard to understand is its consistency. When you eat a 100 calorie food, you are basing the calorie content on a single serving. If you eat two servings, your caloric intake increases to 200 calories. Three servings increase your caloric intake to 300 calories, four servings to 400 calories, and so on. GI rating does not operate in the same manner. When you consume a food with a GI rating of four, the rating remains four regardless of the servings. However, your body will react to consuming more even though the number does not change. Four servings of a high GI food will spike your blood glucose level higher, though the GI rating remains steady.

Do not assume that because a food is generally considered healthy it will have a low GI. This is the thing about eating based on the GI rating of foods. It is a complex concept that does not fall in line with many of the things we know about eating healthy. For instance, pumpkin and parsnips, two extremely healthy vegetables, rank high in the GI rating system. These foods are low in carbohydrates, even though they rank high on the GI scale, so they are perfectly acceptable to eat, even when following a low GI diet. They contain a lot of micronutrients and provide too many benefits to avoid.

The same is true in reverse. There are foods that rank low on the GI rating scale that should not be eaten in excess. For instance, white pasta has a low GI rating, but contains a high number of carbohydrates which play a significant role in weight gain. Its GI rating is low because the un-gelatinized starch is trapped in a network of protein. This is a fancy way of describing gluten.

IS A LOW GI DIET A LOW-CARB DIET?

Though low carbohydrate diets have some similarities to low GI diets, there are differences. You cannot achieve the same affects following a low-carb diet as you can on a GI diet. Low-carb diets produce speedy weight loss because insulin levels are lowered throughout the day. Fat is used as the source of the body's fuel, which is the same as the low GI diet. However, proponents of low GI diets believe low-carb diets are too restrictive and are not practical for long-term results. There are also concerns about the increase in saturated fats on the most popular low-carb diets.

Following a low GI diet is easy and provides a variety of food options. It will take some time to adjust to eating and you will likely refer to your rating chart frequently at first, but you will eventually get the hang of it.

Fruits and Vegetables on a Low GI Diet

Fruits and vegetables are sometimes the toughest challenge on the low GI diet. If you are new to eating healthy, it might be hard to accept some fruits and vegetables should be eaten in moderation. Do not allow yourself to stress about the rules on a low GI diet at first. Swapping any fruit or vegetable for a processed food is a positive change. Over time you can begin to make more exact changes within your newly improved diet.

There are a few general rules to follow in terms of GI rating and fruits and vegetables. Fruits grown in temperate climates, such as apples, pears, and citrus, as well as stone fruits, such as plums, peaches, and nectarines, all have low GI ratings. Tropical fruits have higher ratings, but they are low in carbohydrates. Bananas are starchy and known for their high ranking on the GI scale. Leafy greens are so low on the GI they do not even register. Starchy vegetables, such as corn and potatoes rank fairly high. Yams are one of the lower ranking potatoes, so choose those ahead of red or yellow potatoes. Pumpkins, carrots, beets, and peas all have low ratings and should be enjoyed frequently.

Most people would expect cereal and bread to rank high on the GI scale, but there are options that have a reasonable ranking. Breads made from legume or chickpea flours are much lower, as are cereals that contain psyllium husks. It is also possible to add your own psyllium powder to control blood sugar spikes. Pasta can be problematic, so substitute buckwheat, cellophane, or rice noodles for traditional white pasta. Avoid refined flour products whenever possible and look for hidden refined flour in cereals, crackers, and snack foods.

Another option for lowering the overall GI ranking of a dish is to combine it with legumes or lentils. The boosted fiber lowers the blood sugar spike and allows you to fill up faster on fewer calories. Food pairing is a great way to eat a variety of foods, but keep your GI issues in check. Pair bananas, a high GI fruit, with peanut butter and spread peanut butter or hummus on bagels and toast. Also remember to include healthy fats, such as nuts and olive oil in your diet, as well as organic low-fat dairy or fortified nut milks.

Eating based on GI ranking takes some getting used to, but the GI ratings scale is a helpful tool for choosing foods. As you continue to make healthy changes in your diet, refine your food choices based on GI. If you love bananas and pineapples, use them to replace packaged snacks and salty foods. Once you have adjusted to healthier eating, swap out the bananas and pineapples for apples and pears. You do not have to eliminate the high GI foods completely, but you should treat them as you would indulgences. Over time, low GI eating enables you to lose weight, balance your blood sugar levels, and boost the overall health of your diet. It is a great way to alter your diet and learn to eat healthier.

Chapter 3 - What to Include in Your New Diet

All of the information about the foods that can harm you and the ingredients you need to avoid can feel overwhelming. Too often people are left feeling as if there is nothing safe to eat, but nothing could be further from the truth. There are plenty of foods to eat, even if you have decided to eliminate most of what causes problems. The key is learning the benefits of certain foods and then finding ways to fit those foods into your diet.

Sometimes changing your perspective is the best way to improve your diet and your overall health. Instead of viewing changes as painful and focused on elimination, look at them from a different point of view. See the changes as an opportunity to add new things to your diet. Eliminating dangerous foods prevents disease, but adding food can do just as much good. Some foods boost health and actually interfere with the development or progression of diseases. When you view your lifestyle changes from a place of adding abundance and health to your diet, it will be easier to cope with the difference.

It is also important to note that adding foods to your diet makes it easier to eliminate the bad stuff. When you load up your menu with healthy, beneficial food, there is less room left on your plate and in your stomach for the unhealthy food. Your focus is on trying new things and you feel full, so you rarely worry about all of the foods you are giving up or no longer enjoying.

If necessary, make your changes gradually. Jumping into something new can backfire. It is better to make small changes over time and stick with them than to jump in and revamp your entire diet, only to return to the same poor eating habits in a month or two. There are no rules about changing your diet, as long as you are always moving in the direction of health. Even small changes can help you in the long-run, so no matter how long it takes, be patient with your body and with your tastes. Slow, gradual change is always better than no change at all.

So, where you do begin when you are ready to make diet changes? It can be tempting to rush out to the supermarket and restock your pantry with all new healthy foods. If you are this motivated, go for it! Just make sure you do not over buy and get stuck tossing a bunch of foods. Remember, fresh, unprocessed foods have a shorter shelf life than many of the foods you are giving up. Buy only enough for a few days or a week so you do not waste food.

If you are overwhelmed by all of the choices you can add to your healthier eating plan, you should begin with a few sample foods. It takes time to learn about healthy foods and figure out how to prepare these healthy options, so take your time. You can begin with these foods and build from here. Incorporating the following foods into your new style of eating gives you a great base from which to begin your healthy foods journey.

HEALTHY DRINKS

Drinks are one of the trickiest aspects of eating healthy. What we have learned throughout our lives might not be as accurate as we once believed. Ask the average person and they are likely to tell you milk and fruit juices are healthy. Luckily, most people understand soda is the worst of all beverage choices, but too few realize that fruit juices can be nearly as dangerous and that milk might also cause a threat.

The average fruit juice is packed with sugar. Some juices feature only natural sugars. The important thing to know about these natural juices is that they are not low calorie or diet foods, but they are convenient substitutes when you cannot eat regular fruit. Fruit juices that are made purely from fresh fruit and no added ingredients are healthy alternatives when eating a piece of whole fruit is not an option.

Unfortunately, not all fruit juices are made the same and marketing can fool even the savviest of shoppers. Fruit juices containing anything other than pure fruit are likely packed with added sugar. There might also be dyes and preservatives included in the drinks. When choosing fruit juices, which should be consumed sparingly, you should read the ingredient label closely and opt for juices made only from pure fresh fruit.

Coconut Water

Another problematic beverage is the sports drink. These drinks are intended to help people rebalance electrolytes and rehydrate, particularly after intense physical activity. Unfortunately, the average person consuming sports drinks is not participating in intense activity. And worse, these drinks also contain dyes and other dangerous ingredients. A healthy alternative to sports drinks is coconut water.

Coconut water is a natural alternative to sports drinks, soda, and other sugar-laden beverages. Those who do not like the taste of pure water or who want to mix up their flavors a bit should try coconut water. It has a sweet, slightly meaty taste and can be flavored with natural fruit juices for something different. In addition to tasting great, it is packed with health benefits.

The reason coconut water is such a great alternative to sports drinks is because it is packed with electrolytes. The purpose of sports drinks after physical activity is to rehydrate and rebalance the body's cells. Coconut water contains magnesium, potassium, sodium, calcium, and phosphorous. Each of these plays an important role in our bodies, so keeping them in balance is necessary for good health. Coconut water helps you do this without preservatives or excess calories, making it a healthy choice.

Coconut water has also been proven to lower blood pressure by as much as 70%. People suffering from high blood pressure can drink coconut water first thing in the morning to replenish after a night of not eating. This balances electrolytes and keeps blood pressure in check all day. Coconut water is also low in sugar and contains no high fructose corn syrup. Coconut water helps improve the health of your skin from the inside out and helps heal acne scars. It is a great choice for people who want to lose weight because it is low in calories and contains a lot of fiber. There is also evidence that coconut water is beneficial for curing and preventing kidney stones, balancing pH in blood, treating cholera, preventing acid reflux, aiding digestion, improving circulation, and boosting the immune system. There are even instances in which coconut water was given intravenously as a quick fix for dehydration.

Pomegranate Juice

Pomegranate juice is an excellent alternative to other high sugar, processed fruit juices. It is important to choose pomegranate juice that is natural. If possible, prepare your own from pomegranates and mix with other pure fruit juice, such as blueberry or apple. It can also be blended with sparking water for a carbonated soda alternative.

Pomegranate juice does contain a lot of natural sugar, so health experts recommend drinking it in combination with a salad or oatmeal. However, pomegranate does not cause blood sugar to spike like some sugars, so you do not have to worry about the increase and the plummet. It is a great juice alternative for diabetics, as long as they do not overdo it.

In addition to being a great alternative to other fruit juices and soda, pomegranate juice offers a variety of health benefits. Many health experts consider pomegranate a powerful cancer fighter. Studies show pomegranate juice is capable of destroying breast cancer cells and possibly preventing them from forming in the first place. There is also evidence that it may inhibit the growth of lung cancer cells and prostate cancer. It also keeps PSA levels stable. Studies show men undergoing prostate cancer treatment needed less treatment when consuming pomegranate juice during the course of their treatment.

In addition to prevention of cancer, pomegranate juice also prevents cartilage deterioration, plaque buildup in the arteries, and Alzheimer's disease. Studies have shown it lowers LDL and raises HDL cholesterol, and lowers blood pressure by about 5%. Consumption while pregnant protects the neonatal brain during development and there is even evidence pomegranate juice prevents dental plaque build-up. Incidentally, this prevention of dental plaque likely coincides with the prevention of plaque in the arteries, since many studies show a link between heart disease and plaque buildup. What reduces one type of plaque in the body often helps other plaque-related issues.

Green Tea

Green tea is one of the healthiest beverages you can drink and people should be drinking it every single day. Green tea contains caffeine, so those sensitive to the stimulant will not want to overdo it. However, if you have been drinking coffee for years and you are looking for a caffeinated alternative, you cannot find a better choice than green tea. (Black tea does contain caffeine and it has a number of health benefits, as do all teas, but green in the king of healthy teas).

Green tea is one of the few foods that even the most skeptical of Western medicine practitioners can agree is a natural health miracle. It is filled with antioxidants. Antioxidants search for and eliminate free radicals from the body. Free radicals play a role in the development of cancer, blood clots, and artherosclerosis. There are many sources of antioxidants, but green tea is one of the best. It undergoes minimal processing, so the antioxidants are more concentrated than other teas.

There is some debate over how much green tea is enough. Studies conducted in Asia show higher consumption levels are ideal. One study that included 500 Japanese women with breast cancer showed that green tea consumption reduced the risk of recurrence. Chinese studies have shown similar results with stomach, prostate, pancreatic, esophageal, and colorectal cancers. A study including patients with a high risk of lung cancer showed that high consumption of specifically green tea reduced the risk of cancer development by nearly 20%.

Green tea is great for heart health and is the perfect beverage for those with a desire to lose weight. It is a low calorie drink and a diuretic. Some dieters choose green tea supplements, but the best option is drinking pure green tea. The liquid gives you a feeling of fullness and flushes your system of toxins and water retention. Make sure you are choosing pure green tea beverages when shopping because there are products on the market proclaiming the benefits of tea, but loaded with sugar or artificial sweeteners.

Though you do not want to overdo it with fruit juices, it is easy to see why fresh, unprocessed, unaltered fruit juices are a great alternative to juices and other beverages containing high fructose corn syrup. Green tea is also a great alternative and you are free to drink as much as you like. If you want to enjoy a flavorful beverage in addition to the eight glasses of water you should drink every day, and you are interested in consuming beverages that offer a myriad of health benefits, consider one of these alternatives.

LEAFY GREENS

Leafy greens are one of the best foods you can eat, but they take some getting used to. Some people still remember having to clean their plates of spinach as children or they recall the bitter taste of dark greens in salads. If their taste buds have grown accustomed to the void-of-nutrient bland taste of iceberg lettuce, it will take some time to adjust to the potent taste of darker lettuces. Regardless what your excuses have been up until now concerning leafy greens, you need to incorporate them into your diet.

All leafy greens are beneficial, but there are three you need to add to your diet as soon as possible.

Spinach

A serving of spinach provides almost one-fifth of the recommended daily allowance of fiber. It contains flavonoids, which provide anti-cancer benefits that prevent cell division in the stomach and skin. It is also believed to prevent prostate cancer. It offers relief from inflammation, which also can affect the development of cancer and a variety of other chronic diseases. It is also packed with antioxidants, vitamins A and K, and minerals.

Kale

Kale is the king of health foods. It is actually a member of the cruciferous vegetable family, but is included with the leafy greens listed here because of its appearance and uses. If you only add one thing to improve your diet, make it kale. It is a great diet food with only 36 calories per cup. It is packed with fiber and prevents constipation, lowers blood sugar, and aids digestion. It is packed with antioxidants and offers anti-inflammatory benefits. Many believe kale is one of the best foods you can eat for cancer prevention and healing. Its high fiber content lowers blood pressure and helps with detoxification. It also has a high sulfur content, which is detoxifying. Finally, kale is high in vitamins K, A, and C.

Swiss Chard

Swiss chard has sturdy green leaves veined with color and colorful stalks. Like kale and spinach, it is packed with antioxidants. It provides vitamins E and C, beta-carotine, zinc, and lutein. Its fiber content helps regulate blood sugar and plays a role in cancer prevention. It is a great source of calcium, which makes it an ideal food for vegans. It also promotes brain health, hair health, vision health, and blood health.

Regardless of your dietary needs, leafy greens are a great addition. If you are still not willing to choke down forkfuls of green leaves, consider blending them into smoothies. A handful of kale or spinach mixed with fruits in a blender is unnoticeable to your taste buds, but your body still benefits.

Brassicas

Brassicas are actually part of the cruciferous vegetable category, which they share with kale and collard greens, but for our purposes we will separate them from the leafy greens. Brassicas include cauliflower, broccoli, Brussels sprouts, and cabbage. When people think of vegetables they might have struggled to enjoy as children, members of the brassica family often come to mind. Finding ways to fit these foods into our diets is important because they are actually super foods. Science has shown that brassicas play a powerful role in reducing risk and managing the progression of many serious diseases.

Those at risk for cancer should begin eating brassicas on a daily basis. All vegetables provide vitamins and minerals, but brassicas feature glucosinolates. This compound eliminates carcinogens from the body before they can damage cells. Some doctors believe it also prevents healthy cells from converting to malignant cells. The vegetables are most commonly believed to play a role in the prevention of breast, colorectal, lung, and prostate cancers.

In addition to cancer, eating brassicas can also reduce the risk for heart disease and stroke. Most researchers believe this is because of their high vitamin C and beta-carotene content. Studies show a 4% reduction in coronary heart disease risk and a 6% reduction in the risk of stroke as a result of daily consumption of fruits and vegetables with high vitamin C content. It is also believed that brassicas reduce the risk of vision problems, especially cataracts, because of their lutein content. A study showed a 50% reduction in the need for cataract surgery for people eating just one serving per week of brassicas!

Brassicas can be a tough dining challenge for those who are just transitioning to healthy eating. It is important to find a few go-to recipes you enjoy, so you are sure to consume the recommended amounts. Often, simple preparations with spices are the best way to go. However, if you have a strong aversion, you can add brassicas to pasta dishes or casseroles. When chopped and paired with sauces, even the most unlikable foods become palatable. Remember, if there is one food in a particular category you just are unable to tolerate, you can up your consumption of other foods from the same category. Hate Brussels sprouts? You can always eat broccoli and cabbage more frequently. You will not enjoy all of the benefits Brussels sprouts offer, but you will come close.

Quinoa

Quinoa is usually found in the supermarket near the rice and pasta products, but it is not a grain. It is related to the spinach family and is actually a seed. Quinoa is a complete protein, which means it contains all nine of the essential amino acids that are considered the building blocks of muscles. Quinoa is similar to rice or couscous when cooked, with a subtle flavor and fluffy texture.

In addition to offering the essential amino acids, quinoa is also high in magnesium, fiber, manganese, and copper. It lowers blood pressure, cleanses the colon, and provides antioxidants that help eliminate free radicals associated with cancer development. It is also high in calcium, phosphorous, iron, and zinc. Some believe eating quinoa helps manage or prevent insulin resistance and diabetes, breast cancer, and artherosclerosis. It is gluten free, so it is the ideal substitute for those who are unable to digest grains and it acts as a pre-biotic providing healthy bacterium for the intestines.

Quinoa is the ideal food for those transitioning to a life of healthy eating, but it should also be included in an ideal diet plan. When possible swap pasta and white rice for quinoa. It makes a great base for stir fry dishes and can be combined with roasted vegetables for a meal or served as a side dish to accompany other foods. It can even be served cold in salads with raw fruits and vegetables.

FRUIT

Fruit is one of the complex healthy foods in existence. It is a great alternative to processed sugary snacks and provides a great pick-me-up if you need a boost. However, it still contains sugar and too much of it is too much, regardless of its form. Your best bet is to use fruit as a transitional tool and then err on the side of caution. If your diet is packed with unhealthy foods currently and you are not yet ready to take on the health powerhouses, fruit is an option that even the unhealthiest of eaters can handle. Once your diet is moving in the right direction, you can begin to use fruit more sparingly. You can also choose fruits that contain less sugar and provide the highest amount of health benefits. Two are standouts in this category.

Berries

Raspberries rank high on the healthy fruit list. They are a low calorie food with only 64 calories per cup and contain amazing amounts of protein and fiber per gram. They feature potassium, calcium, carotenoids, and antioxidants. Health experts believe berries help slow cancer growth and prevent cancer from developing in the first place. A 2010 study showed that mice that were fed berries for three months experienced a reduction in inflammation and inhibited tumor growth.

Blueberries contain more antioxidants than any other fruit. This helps eliminate free radicals and lowers a person's risk for cancer. They are low in calories, so they are a sweet alternative to high sugar and fat desserts. Studies show blueberries have a positive impact on the urinary tract, vision, brain health, heart disease, and digestion. Mixing raspberries and blueberries in a salad or a blended smoothie is a great way to get double the benefit from your berries.

Cantaloupe

Cantaloupe does not rate as well on the glycemic index as berries, but it is so packed with health benefits, it is worth the extra sugar. It is ideal as a substitute for high sugar cereals, sweets, and snacks because it will satisfy the craving for sweets without going overboard. Cantaloupe is a great source of folate, which is a water-soluble B vitamin. It prevents anemia and keeps the cells of the body healthy. Cantaloupe is high in carotenoids, which reduces a person's risk for cancer and cardiovascular disease. It can also reduce macular degenerations. Cantaloupe is a source of vitamin C and potassium, as well.

Ideally, healthy eaters will treat fruit as a dessert item, but there are certain fruits that can be consumed in higher amounts without the risk of over-consuming calories. Whole fruits, consumed with skin if possible, are your best option because they are highest in fiber. Regardless where you are on your healthy foods journey, you should sample as many different fruits as possible and find ways to fit two to three servings into your daily diet.

Steel Cut Oats

Steel cut oats are another member of the super foods category. It should be noted that steel cut oats and oatmeal are not the same as rolled, instant, or quick cooking oats. The packages of oatmeal that you combine with hot water do not provide the same benefits as steel cut oats. In some cases, they are loaded with sugar and chemicals, so if you do occasionally eat quick or instant oats choose carefully and add your own flavorings.

Steel cut oats are derived from the same plant as instant oats, but they are processed differently. Steel cut oats are not cooked until you cook them. They are a whole grain, so they take longer to cook, but offer a complete grain that has not been altered by processing. They contain protein, minerals, vitamins, and soluble and insoluble fibers. They are great for people trying to lose weight and regulate their digestive system.

The fiber content in steel cut oats provides the most potent health benefits. They have five grams of fiber per quarter cup, two grams of which is insoluble. Insoluble fiber helps balance blood sugar levels and improves cholesterol. It is especially helpful for diabetics because it slows the digestive process and lowers the glycemic boost caused by many foods. Steel cut oats also contain trace amounts of amino acids and iron. The average adult can get 10% of their daily iron requirements from a quarter cup of steel cut oats. They are a great alternative to toast or pastries for breakfast, and they fill you up and provide energy for hours after you have finished eating. Perhaps most appealing of all, they are hearty and comforting during the colder months of the year, especially when paired with cinnamon and nuts.

SPICES

In addition to the whole, fresh foods you should incorporate in your diet, it is also a good idea to add certain spices. This serves two purposes. The first is to help you transition to a healthier diet. When you eliminate many of the unhealthy foods, you will also eliminate salt. Your meals will taste bland and unappetizing because you have grown accustomed to eating salty foods. Spices help make unsalted, fresh food palatable. They also provide a number of health benefits.

If you are struggling with your new diet or you are looking for even more ways to boost the health benefits of what you eat, consider adding these spices to the menu.

Cinnamon

Cinnamon is believed to help control blood sugar and lower bad cholesterol levels. It can be sprinkled on oatmeal, coffee, and toast. Be careful to choose pure cinnamon and not cinnamon sugar when shopping.

Turmeric

Turmeric is lesser known than cinnamon and its taste might take a bit of getting used to. However, it is well worth it and considered the superstar of spices. It has a number of anti-inflammatory qualities and many believe it reduces risk of cancer. It is used to flavor savory dishes, such as chicken, eggs, or vegetables.

Cayenne Pepper

Cayenne pepper is a potent spice that adds heat to foods. It contains capsaicin, which has been proven to be a strong anti-inflammatory ingredient. In addition to reducing the risk of diseases associated with inflammation, cayenne pepper is also helpful for reducing the swelling and pain from arthritis or injuries.

Garlic

Garlic is available in a variety of forms, including whole bulbs, crushed, powdered, and sliced. It contains vitamin C, some of the B vitamins, and sulfur compounds. It is effective for reducing blood pressure and triglycerides. It is also believed to contain a variety of cancer fighting properties.

Ginger

Ginger is considered one of the healthiest spices and its sweet-spicy taste is very pleasing to many people. It eases nausea and indigestion and boosts the immune system. Some believe it is also helpful for relieving cold and flu symptoms. Ginger has antioxidant and anti-inflammatory benefits, making it an effective food for preventing and treating a variety of serious illnesses and conditions.

RECOMMENDED READING

During my research on the how to age naturally and how to keep your brain healthy, I came across these books, which may also be helpful to you. You check them out on my site here:

www.YourNaturalYouth.com/Recommended

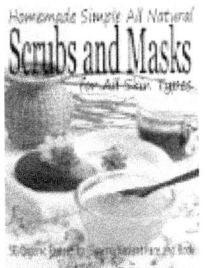

Homemade Simple all Natural Scrubs and Masks: Healthy, Quick and Easy Recipes for Face and Body Exfoliating Scrubs with Nourishing Facial Masks for Different Skin Types

This is a collection of 25 Face Masks and 25 Scrubs Recipes which are for different skin types and use of these recipes will bring back the 25 in you.

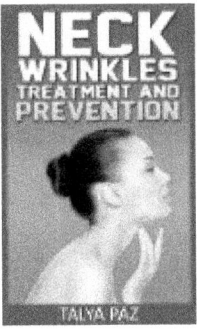

Neck wrinkles treatment and prevention (neck wrinkles, anti-aging, skin care, cosmetics, beauty, aromatherapy, essential oils)

This book will give you all the important information to delay the aging of your skin especially your neck and décolleté area. You will be provided with the necessary tips on how to delay the appearance of wrinkles, how to treat existing ones, how to treat loose neck muscles and how to make the skin look pretty, delicate and smooth.

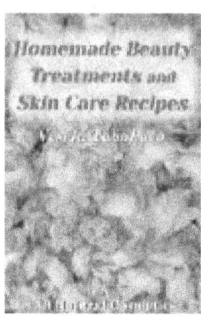

Homemade Beauty Treatments and Skin Care Recipes (All Natural Cosmetics)

A collection of some of the best skin care recipes, as well as various tips and advice on how to have a gorgeous and healthy-looking hair.

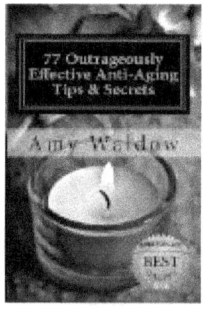

Anti-Aging Book: 77 Outrageously Effective Anti-aging Tips & Secrets – Natural Anti-Aging Strategies and Longevity Secrets Proven to Reverse the Aging ... Tips, Recipes, and Remedies Series

This book contains 77 simple, yet very successful, and exceptionally powerful tips you can take daily to delay the natural aging process.

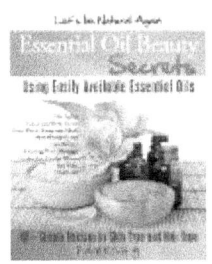

Essential Oils Beauty Secrets: Make Beauty Products at Home for Skin Care, Hair Care, Lip Care, Nail Care and Body Massage for Glowing, Radiant Skin and Shiny Hairs.

This is a compilation of only the most effective and natural recipes to make every women feel and look beautiful. In no time, you will be able to prepare a natural, organic beauty product at home and at a fraction of a cost of conventional chemical products.

About the Author

Dr. Patel is the founder of www.YourNaturalYouth.com and a board certified family physician who also specializes in wound care. He has practiced as a physician for 10 years and has witnessed the ups and downs of our medical system. After frustration with dealing with bureaucratic hospitals and insurance companies,

Dr. Patel concluded that the only way any health care system will improve and be sustainable is if the system puts the power back into the patients' hands and make them feel responsible and educated about their own health.

He has diligently studied the core reasons as to why people get ill and feel chronically fatigued. After several years of research, he has gone to the internet to empower patients. The internet is full of false and misleading medical information from non-physicians. He believes that it is due time that patients have access to physicians online (from all specialties, led by a trusted physician) who can provide them with reliable unbiased information. This will be a reputable multi-specialty online community of board certified physicians they can trust and a place they can call their online medical home. Does one truly believe they can address all their concerns in a 15 minute visit with their primary care doctor that occurs a few times per year? Dr. Patel and his colleagues are here to fill the gap.

Dr. Patel has worn several hats. He has worked as a solo physician, a wound care physician, an immediate care physician and has also played a consultant role for several medical organizations. He prides himself in keeping medicine honest and simple wherein, there is room for both western medicine and other types of therapies in our healthcare system. One of his goals is to spread as much truthful and reliable medical information to all of those that feel that they are not getting their fair share from the medical system and are dealing with the realities of aging.

Dr. Patel is a member of the American Academy of Family Physicians, American Medical Association, American Osteopathic Association, and the American Academy of Anti-Aging Medicine. He attended University of Illinois Urbana-Champaign where he received a bachelor's in Microbiology and completed medical school at Chicago College of Osteopathic Medicine. He went on to complete his medical residency training in an esteemed community hospital in the suburbs of Chicago and also has received additional specialty certification in wound care for the aging population.

When Dr. Patel takes his doctor hat off, he enjoys spending time with his family, playing tennis, golf, basketball, traveling and assisting local and international charities in raising funds.

Get connected with Dr. Patel on Google+ and Facebook.

www.ingramcontent.com/pod-product-compliance
Lightning Source LLC
Chambersburg PA
CBHW070820290526

45795CB00002B/778